FOREVER STAGE IV

Forever Stage IV

One Woman's Journey with
ALK+ Lung Cancer

Millie Lintell

MERIPOINT BOOKS

Contents

I pray that you may have strength to comprehend with all the holy ones what is the breadth and length and height and depth, and to know the love of Christ that surpasses knowledge, so that you may be filled with all the fullness of God.

Ephesians 3:18-19

To Bill

Introduction

*A*ll the things in this world are gifts of
God, created for us, to be the means by
which we can come to know him better,
love him more surely, and serve him more
faithfully.

— St. Ignatius of Loyola

This little book tells the story of my journey thus
far with ALK+ lung cancer. It is my sincere wish
that you who read it may benefit from it whether or
not cancer has snuck into your life.

ML

September 2023

x

Chapter I
2020 Vision

You ought not to cure eyes without head,
Or head without body,
So you should not treat body without soul.
—Plato

One misty November afternoon, I drove down the road when I realized that I couldn't see clearly out of my right eye. I blinked rapidly several times yet it didn't help. I wiped my glasses at a traffic stop. That didn't help either. My eye couldn't focus on anything. I decided to return home.

My eyesight had been getting perceptively worse since the summer. Little things were becoming difficult such as seeing the hands on the kitchen clock over the stove or seeing our cat in a distance. Soon, everything viewed through my right eye was a blur even with my trusted eyeglasses on.

I went to my eye doctor. He discovered a fast growing sub-capsular cataract. He told me this typically happens as the result of a past injury. That seemed odd as I had never injured my eye and I was young for cataracts. He assured me that there was a solution: a well-established surgical procedure to replace the lens. I would have two surgeries, first the clouded eye, second the other, both scheduled in early 2020. I didn't look forward to cataract surgery, however, I was cautiously optimistic about the outcome. If all went according to plan, I would have clear vision for the first time in my memory. To be able to see without glasses was a dream. The timing was perfect as well. I had plans to fly to England in late May to walk the Dales Way with a friend. I would be able to enjoy the English countryside with new eyes.

I met with my eye surgeon in early February. He mentioned the new flu that everyone was discussing, Covid-19. Initially, I shrugged it off. He looked at me seriously and said, "This is a *pandemic*. We need to get these surgeries done." We scheduled the first for late February.

News of Covid-19 started to saturate the internet, the newspapers, and everyone's conversations. I didn't pay too much attention to it as I personally was struggling with my eyesight. The first surgery went well and I was left with one eye 20/20 and the other 20/300. I had to endure this for two weeks—I felt I could push through. I couldn't wear my old glasses. They were frameless and it was impossible to remove one lens. My ophthalmologist had given me a contact lens to wear in the 20/300 eye. I hadn't worn contacts for twenty years and it was difficult to adjust. I struggled with it and found it impossible. The two weeks were head-ache inducing and I stayed close to home.

Early in the morning on the Ides of March, we arrived at Langley Air Force Base for the second surgery. The process was similar to the first. The next day I went to my follow-up appointment. As we drove from the gate to the clinic, I noticed that the roads and parking lot were eerily empty. My husband and I navigated the hallways to the eye clinic, and the building echoed. We didn't encounter anyone. We entered the clinic. I looked around noting that all seats were empty. A technician behind the reception area beckoned me over at once. He signed me in, immediately after which my doctor called me to the exam room. After he examined my new lenses and determined that all was well, he told me that my eye surgery was the last that he would be able to perform for the foreseeable future. All non-Covid-19 and non-life-threatening medical procedures were officially on hold. This clinic and every other medical clinic were closed. He explained that he did not know when he would resume seeing his eye patients.

I was shocked and asked him about those who had only one eye corrected. He said that there was nothing he could do for them. They'd have to wait for their second eye surgery until the pandemic lifted. I then asked him about cancer patients. What happens to them? He explained that they'll have to wait for their treatments until things open up again.

That is when it hit me: Covid-19 was real. The lock-downs and shutdowns were real. We were about to experience something I had never even imagined could happen. To confirm my feelings of dread, every day brought news of more and more of the world shutting down.

I tried not to dwell on it too much. I had new eyes, I could see so much that I never saw before, and I was looking forward to this fabulous walking trip with my good friend in late May. I was confident that everything would be back to normal by then.

We had been planning this trip for over a year. It was going to be my unofficial Moms' graduation trip. Our children were launched, and this phase of our jobs as stay-at-home moms was done. We wanted to celebrate. In the fall of 2019, we booked the B&Bs. We bought the necessary gear. My eldest daughter, who had a foreboding about my plans, made sure I had the correct hiking boots and socks

—both critical for long-distance walking. She also insisted I have a GPS monitoring system with me. I found a good waterproof jacket. In early January, we decided to hire a sherpa to transport our baggage. The only thing left to do was to buy our plane tickets. This was when things became dicey.

It started with Italy. I wasn't concerned. Italy is Italy. Then other European countries announced that their borders, too, were closed. Overnight, no travelers were being allowed in or out. Neither my friend nor I wanted to face the reality of what this meant for our adventure. One-by-one each British B&B notified me that our reservations were cancelled. All of the hotels and accommodations in Great Britain were under lockdown and no one would be allowed to stay in them until who knows when. It was clear; our walking tour was no more.

Then it happened here. My youngest daughter was home for her spring break from university when U.S. authorities imposed a nation-wide lockdown which severely restricted everyone's movements beyond their homes. It was to be two weeks of complete isolation throughout the country to flatten the curve, the rate at which the Covid-19 infections spread. Students could not return to campus until the lockdown was lifted.

Two weeks, I thought, we could do this. My husband and I sheltered at home. I figured that we would now have time to read books from our growing collection of must-reads. My youngest daughter and another university student moved into our home to complete their semester via the suddenly ubiquitous *zoom*. The four of us and our little green-eyed cat formed what was called a "pod." My other two adult children hunkered down in their homes, likewise isolated from the world. Their lifelines were zoom and their phones.

We left our house only for specific purposes, mainly grocery shopping which I did alone to minimize our exposure. I continued my outdoor walks with close friends, maintaining the required six foot distance. During these outdoor treks, I stretched my eyes as far as they could go. After all, I had a new view of the world. My husband continued to go into the office as he was literally the only person in the building.

Governments are not known for efficiency, and true to form, the two-week lockdown stretched into months. We remained in isolation through March, April, May, and June. Finally, restrictions lifted a smidgen in June, allowing our university house guest the chance to move to her own apartment. Things were looking better, still highly unusual, but better. There was a tentative sense of relief in the air.

After three months, the first thing I wanted to do was to go to my favorite little shops and see familiar people. I wanted to go to the library and to church without being required to sign up on a list. Many of these things were still not possible in June as there was still a sense of tentativeness. We were eager to reconnect with our peers, friends, and family but we weren't sure what was safe and what was not. We were bombarded with conflicting opinions. Nevertheless, hope was in the air and I was confident that normalcy would return.

Although cancelled this year, my friend and I were already making plans to hike the Dales Way in perhaps the following year, so we continued our rigorous training walks.

One Friday morning in June, we decided to walk around the entire Jamestown Island, about 9 miles, a lovely walk free of cars as the roads were still closed. We had to walk faster than usual because of time constraints. I felt up to the challenge. My friend was a far more accomplished long-distance walker than I, but I had been able to keep up with her during previous strenuous walks.

We purposefully plunged forward for the first six miles. All was well. The trees were beautiful and I could see details and color nuances that I had never seen before. My friend and I chatted for a few miles and then fell into silence as we typically did.

As we continued along the path, I suddenly felt heavy, and my heart began to race. Not too concerned, I took a few deep breaths. Then I noticed that even though I thought I was moving as quickly as before, my legs were fighting forward motion. It was like walking in molasses. I was soon far behind my friend. My heart pounded. I could feel every beat. My legs struggled. I wasn't making progress. My breathing became increasingly labored. I focused on the ground, forcing my legs to continue forward.

My friend was by now a small figure in the distance. She stopped for a moment and glanced back, looking for me. Time was ticking. We had to make it back to the car. I pushed as hard as I could. Forward, heart pounding, deep breath, forward. At last the pavement changed and I knew that the car was within reach. My friend waited for me in a shady area as I finally caught up. She looked at me and realized that I was struggling. I waved off her concern. The car was within sight and I was almost there. Those last 500 feet were long, but I trudged forward until at last I fell upon the hood of my car. After a few moments, my heart calmed a bit and I laughed at my silliness for not being able to keep up. This was a strange fluke.

A week later my friend left town for awhile, but I continued to take short walks several times a week with other friends. All was fine. Then in early July, as I started a leisurely stroll with a neighbor, I realized I couldn't go on. I explained that I was just a little tired, that's all. In reality this simple five-minute exertion exhausted me and once I got inside, I made a beeline for the sofa and told the house to let me rest for awhile. From that point on, day after day, my energy levels continued to drop. I cancelled all of my walks, and everything, actually.

I couldn't get beyond this exhaustion. By mid-July, I no longer did anything during the day. Now, in addition to the exhaustion, my heart beat erratically at random times for increasingly longer intervals no matter what I did. I assumed that it was all tied together as an after-effect of the stresses of the lockdown. I decided I needed rest and vitamins, especially B-12. Sleeping, however, became difficult because my heart raced whenever I lay down. My husband, thinking it might be due to low blood pressure, bought a blood pressure measuring device. My blood pressure was in the normal zone.

One morning, I realized that I couldn't smell my shower soap, and I couldn't taste my morning coffee. I was still able to breathe, so I dismissed the notion that I had Covid, even though a tiny voice in the back of my head kept whispering, "maybe you have Covid…" Covid tests were not yet available. I tried to ignore that little whisper.

The last week of July rolled around. My husband had to go on a week-long trip. I told him that I'd be fine, I just needed rest. Naturally, as soon as he left my breathing became labored and my heart now beat so hard that I was no longer able to stand easily or sit up for very long. When I did sit up, I had to have my knees pressed against my chest. This was a balancing act on the tall kitchen stool, but I managed.

It was now only my youngest daughter and I in the house. She took care of the meals but I could no longer eat and breathe simultaneously so I lost interest in eating. Nevertheless, I still believed this was something I could get over on my own. I took more Vitamin C and B-12. My daughter was not as sure and didn't want me to die in my sleep so she put the dinner bell by my bed to ring if I needed her.

Then on the last Thursday of July, my son came to visit. He saw me on the sofa and told me directly I had to see a doctor. I politely declined explaining that it wasn't necessary. He wouldn't let it go. He became insistent. There was resolve in his voice and in the way he looked at me that caused me to re-think my determination to manage on my own. On Friday, I finally relented and he drove me to a local Urgent Care. It was in the nick of time.

They ruled out Covid immediately to my great relief. They hooked me up to an EKG[1] and found that it was far worse than I expected—my heart was failing—sudden cardiac death was close.

My son rushed me to the emergency room at Langley Air Force Base. He helped me out of the car and steered me toward the only entrance available to us: a long tent tunnel that had to be traversed

---

[1] Electrocardiogram

before reaching a Covid-screening checkpoint. Our heretofore swift flight toward emergency care was abruptly halted by two women seated behind a table with thermometers, masks, and paperwork in front of them. One asked why we were there, and after approving our reason, she took our temperatures. After passing that initial screening, the other looked at a Covid symptom checklist and asked whether either of us were experiencing symptoms. Leaning heavily on my son, with my breathing capability diminished by my mask, I was clearly unable to represent myself. My son managed to convince them that I needed to be seen immediately. They relented but told him he couldn't accompany me and they were not authorized to do anything more. Luckily, he finally managed to convince them to let him take me to the triage nurse.[2]

At the intake station, they put me in a wheelchair, asked questions and then told my son to leave the building immediately. He wasn't allowed in the waiting room or anywhere else.

As a nurse whisked me away, my son reluctantly left and walked across the burning pavement of the tree-barren, empty parking lot to his car. It was a hot, humid July day, but there he waited.

---

[2] In retrospect, the whole process would have been easier if upon seeing the screening table, I just fainted and plunked down to the floor.

Back inside the air-conditioned hospital, they gave me aspirin in case I had a blockage. After an x-ray, they found that my right lung had completely collapsed and the pleural lining, which should have been flat, was plumped full of fluid. This swelling was squeezing my femoral artery and displaced my heart causing it to fail.[3] I had to be hospitalized.

I was thoroughly baffled about the collapsed lung. What caused my lung to collapse? And what was a pleural lining? Why did it fill with fluid? I thought back to my walks and the increasing difficulties I had had. How long had my lung been collapsing? Again, I thought the whole predicament was odd and couldn't for the life of me figure out how I managed to do this. I knew answers would come soon enough and at this point I was relieved that someone was going to fix me.

I rested in a curtained-off area across from the staff station and listened as the doctor pleaded with various hospitals to find a bed for me. As I learned later, this was another consequence of the Covid lockdowns. Hospitals did not have their usual number of beds. They were required to reserve one-third of their beds for potential Covid patients, but for the most part remained empty.

At one point, the doctor popped in to tell me that she found a bed at Bethesda Naval Hospital—

---

[3] No wonder I couldn't walk.

four hours away in Maryland. I thought to myself, "Hmmmm." It seemed far.

Fortunately, she wasn't satisfied with this and told me she'd keep trying. The clock ticked on as I dozed and my son waited in his car. In the early evening the doctor returned with the happy news that she negotiated a bed for me at Portsmouth Naval Hospital, only about 30 miles from Langley. I was relieved. They whisked me off to a waiting ambulance for a ride through the tunnel to Portsmouth and sent a text to my son telling him that he could go home.

I was put into a double-room on the pediatric floor. The bed beside me was empty. All patients had a private room to minimize potential exposure and were placed on any non-Covid floor that had an empty room. Everything was a bit mixed up.

There weren't many patients in the hospital, but there were plenty of medical staff coming and going. The constant attention surprised me. I knew that Portsmouth Hospital was a behemoth but I didn't realize it was also a teaching hospital where medical staff included young interns and residents, who were full of new knowledge and enthusiasm. They seized my case with all of the energy of youth and were determined to discover what was going on with my heart and lungs.

The experience was overwhelming at times. It seemed as though there was an unending stream of technicians to draw blood, or young interns asking the same questions over and over about my medical history which I admit was scanty. And this was before the scans started. My poor body with its limping heart had to undergo many x-rays, ultrasounds, and CT scans. Each time they wheeled in another machine, I daydreamed about taking mega amounts of vitamin C.[4]

They stabilized my heart, and I immediately felt much better. My lung was still collapsed, and there remained a sack of fluid surrounding one lung, but with my heart beating correctly I could breathe with less effort. I felt the danger point had passed and now all that I needed was to get rid of the pleural fluid and re-inflate my lung. I thought this was very do-able. It was a weekend and not many specialists were available. I waited patiently, knowing that I would soon be out and could resume my life.

I turned on the screen next to the bed and flipped through the channels looking for a fun movie. I stopped at an episode of *Twilight* which was new to me. As I was watching, my heart suddenly seized and spazzed out of control. It was worse than ever, and I was rushed to the ICU.

This is why I have tried to prioritize healthy living habits. No one should have to experience

---

[4] Vitamin C is known as a powerful anti-oxidant. It helps cells repair damage due to radiation.

what I did in the ICU where extreme measures were taken to save my life. They were painful, no way around it. For those who like gruesome details, I'll simply say, without anesthesia, they cut through to the pleural that surrounded my lung, inserted a straw, and drew out the fluid which caused my lung to inflate like a balloon popping in reverse, to everyone's surprise. This was not what they expected. I don't know what was more painful: the knife inserted through my ribs to extract the fluid or the rapid lung inflation. But neither of those helped my heart—which was now completely bonkers. With my permission, because of course I was fully conscious throughout all of this, they chemically stopped my heart and restarted it. I'll never forget it. When they finally transferred me out of the ICU and back to a regular room, I was so grateful to be far away from that place. Yet despite all of the testing and scans and now ICU stay, no one told me what was causing all of this.

A day or so later, dark before sunrise, I underwent a PET[5] scan.

Later that morning, the lead doctor on my case brought in a large group of medical students. They gathered at the foot of my bed. I was feeling much better and in good spirits. I sat up and looked at the group, patiently waiting for the usual questions.

---

[5] Positron emission tomography

After saying good morning to me, the doctor turned towards her students and began her briefing by saying that this patient is a Stage IV lung cancer patient.

"What?" I asked loudly.

The doctor turned to me confused, "Didn't anyone tell you?"

I said no.

She turned back to her students. "Everybody, out of the room at once." They left quickly.

She sat down next to me. Previously brusque and efficient, she suddenly seemed human. She looked at me with gentle eyes and told me in a soft voice that they found malignant cells in the pleural fluid and a malignant lesion in my lung. They also found lesions on a rib, in my liver and lymph nodes. The PET scan revealed seven lesions in my brain. The origin of the cancer was in the lung.

"You've never smoked, have you?" She asked me.

I had not. She then explained that the type of lung cancer that I had is non-small cell lung cancer (NSCLC), a fairly common cancer that is slow growing, typically found in non-smokers. In my case, the primary tumor was relatively small and she was surprised that it had metastasized.

"Do you have any questions?"

"What is the prognosis?"

"You have a significant malignant pleural effusion. The primary tumor is inoperable, There is no possibility for radiation. The cancer has spread to your brain in seven areas. If you do nothing at all, then you cannot expect to live beyond three months."

My mind went blank.

"Do you have any other questions?"

"No." I paused for a few seconds, looked at the white board with its colorful scribbled notes detailing my daily status, turned back to her, and said, "Thank you."

She nodded and left the room.

I knew something was dreadfully wrong. My heart was in obvious distress. But cancer, my zodiac sign which I had always been slightly nervous about, was the farthest thing from my mind. Now to hear that my cancer wasn't just "Hey, you have cancer, but it's early so we are going to get ahead of it and you can lead a normal life" cancer. It was a "whoops, surprise! You're one step from the grave" cancer. My demise was to be in as little as three months. This was incredulous to me.

Three months is a meaningful demarcation of time in my family. It was the time we needed to pack up our household before moving to a new location whenever my husband had a permanent change of station during his active duty Air Force days. It would take three months on both ends of a move: three months to pack up and three months to unpack. That was just how we operated. I knew military wives who could organize everything in a single week before a move and then unpack so quickly after their arrival at their new location that they had fresh flowers on the table for dinner that night. For me, it was three months.

After the doctor left, the concept kept cycling through my mind: three months to live. It wasn't enough time. I kept repeating in my mind that I needed far more time to move out of my old life into not another town or place but into an unknown. And this move would be so different because nothing would be coming with me, and no one would be accompanying me. I had to do this completely alone. It was surreal. I couldn't accept that three months was enough time.

While sitting in that hospital room, on that bed, connected to myriad devices, with a mask over my mouth and nose, I needed to think. I didn't want to talk to anyone. I didn't want to read or watch movies. I just wanted to mull over this personally devastating news.

Sometime later one of my favorite nurses came in. She was well-prepared for a thoroughly demoralized patient. I was more sober than she expected. I couldn't afford the luxury of falling apart. I asked her a few questions about lung cancer. She didn't have answers, so she whipped out her phone and started to look them up. We sat on my bed, googling for answers for what seemed like a long time. It was comforting.

Soon it was time to pack up and go home. My stay at this hospital was over.

The medical staff had done all that they could. My heart was stabilized and beating as it should, much of the fluid was drained and my lung was about 70% inflated. I was breathing well. I was still wobbly on my feet but I could walk unassisted. Unfortunately, there was nothing to prevent the fluid from building up again, so I was given an appointment with the pulmonologist the following week to determine how to handle the fluid build-up.

As I was preparing to go, one of the doctors took my husband aside, out of my earshot, and told him to get my affairs in order. He said, "Nobody comes back from where she is. It is very unlikely she'll make it to Thanksgiving."

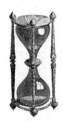

Chapter II
The Plan

I was discharged from the hospital with the diagnosis of metastatic adenocarcinoma of lung origin: the primary tumor being 2.6 centimeters long. The other lesions as noted were located in the brain, rib, liver, and lymph nodes.

The treatment plan called for gamma knife radiation to the brain within two weeks and chemo-therapy to attack the other sites of malignancy afterwards. Neither surgery nor general radiation were possibilities.

The chemo-therapy part of the plan was yet in question. We were awaiting the results of the mutational/molecular testing.

It sounds simple as I write it out, however, it was not. Tired and dazed, I returned home, plopped down on the sofa in the family room, and fell asleep.

That weekend was a blur — I slept through it to slowly regain strength. Family and friends delivered food and flowers and small gifts to cheer me up.

It was impossible to be cheerful. I had to think. I had to work out what came next. I was experiencing a strange combination of regret, incredulousness, and peace. A peculiar duality of thought took over. On the one hand, I wanted to fight to survive. On the other, I wanted to clean up the house, get rid of things, and put everything in order before I died.

In the hospital, after receiving the bad news, I made a list of twenty-one things to do before I died. This list included what we always did to prepare for a move such as filing all paperwork, making sure all tax documentation was in order, tossing old or broken things including clothing and shoes, and updating inventories. The rest of the list was all about tying up loose ends and enjoying a few things that I had been saving for later.

By Monday, I was up and on the phone to begin the round of phone calls to get my treatment started. This was a priority. I had three months.

My primary care provider was first on the list. She set up a case manager for me within the military health system. I touched base with both the oncology practice that the Portsmouth doctors referred me to and the neurosurgeon who would perform the gamma knife procedure. Meanwhile, my husband handled the insurance companies. It took about a week for the referrals and authorizations to leave Portsmouth, so although I called all of these offices, I couldn't set up appointments right away.

My primary care provider told me that I needed to learn as much as possible about this cancer. She recommended starting with two books—both of which introduce integrative strategies for approaching advanced cancer.

The first, *How to Starve Cancer*[6], is one woman's story of her experience with Stage IV cancer in 1994 at the age of 35. She refused to accept a dire prognosis, and instead dove deep into research and studies to find a path to treating her cancer without worsening her situation. The result of her efforts is a metabolic protocol wherein traditional genetic approaches (such as chemotherapy) are combined with the use of off-label medications and the adoption of both dietary and lifestyle changes as an overall strategy for defeating cancer. She summarizes research that was conducted in the 1920s[7] by Dr. Otto Warburg that clearly showed that cancer cells were sugar junkies. This spoke to my

---

[6] McLelland

[7] Otto Warburg was awarded the Nobel Prize in Physiology in 1931 for discovering that cancer cells have damaged mitochondria and produce most of their energy in the cells' cytoplasm, thereby requiring huge amounts of glucose and glutamine.

heart. I had long considered processed sugar as evil and tried to avoid it. Now, I had scientific support.

I liked her overall approach. I felt a combination of standard oncology treatment combined with things that I could do was the best strategy for me.

The author of the second book, *Cancer Secrets*, practices integrative oncology and corroborates much of what the first book suggests. As a medical doctor, he combines conventional medicine (allopathic) with alternative medicine (what he terms holistic or natural). This again was the approach I wanted to take. This author, like the previous one, argues that cancer is mainly a metabolic disease and the result of stresses overtaking our body's ability to cope resulting in harmful inflammation. He, too, references the research of Dr. Warburg and notes more recent research[8] conducted in 2009 that expands upon Dr. Warburg's work to conclude in a nutshell that cancer is all about malfunctioning mitochondria, or the breakdown of mitochondria resulting in the cell's inability to feed itself through normal channels.

Both books were helpful and gave me hope that I could fight this cancer, yet they were emotionally difficult to get through.

---

[8] Seyfried, 2010

The words were easy enough to comprehend. But I wanted there to be a simple solution to this cancer, like the new lens that replaced my cataract-clouded eye. In many medical fields, the experts agree fairly well with one another on how to treat the problem. Not so with cancer, where every case is different and no one knows for certain the absolute correct treatment. We have statistics, we can perform surgery, we have cell-zapping technologies, and we have powerful chemistry. But no doctor can tell the cancer patient, especially the advanced cancer patient, whether the standard protocol is going to kill them or save them. The best they can do is to point to statistics.

Be Your Own Advocate

My primary care doctor told me that I had to be my own advocate from day one, and I jumped into that role immediately. I had to learn about and think deeply about all of the possible approaches to this cancer and make my own decisions. I also had to work with my oncology team to find the right strategy specifically for me. By balancing the treatment options that they recommended with what I know about my body and how it reacts, I could make reasonable decisions about my care.

There were many early obstacles. Insurance, for instance, was more complicated than I anticipated, and because of a mix-up, I wasn't able to make my initial appointments in the time frame set by the Portsmouth doctors. Two weeks would pass before my initial visit with an oncologist; I first saw the brain surgeon in late August.

The theme of my cancer is that *time* is critical. Yet a voice inside of me told me not to make rash decisions, that perhaps this delay is not a terrible thing.[9] While I read and plotted and waited, my husband was busy with his own channels of information.

A week after being discharged from the hospital, a Priority Mail package arrived at our home, not surprising as my husband loves to shop. This package, however, contained something new to our world: a small container of gallium maltolate, a white, reportedly safe powder.[10] The instructions were to measure a precise amount and mix it in

---

[9] Cancer is a tricky business. One shouldn't delay treatment hoping for something better; but then one shouldn't simply, out of desperation, jump at the first treatment suggested. It is incumbent upon the cancer patient to research their condition and the possible treatments or find someone who can do it for them. Many people have advised me to seek a second opinion if and when I have doubts. This I will do, if necessary.

[10] Prior to taking this, I had signed a letter saying that I knew that gallium maltolate has not been approved for any medical use, and I agreed that it could only be used under the supervision of a physician.

water or ice cream or some similar, non-acidic food. I was to take this every morning. I don't eat ice cream so I chose to mix it in water. It had the aroma of strawberry cotton candy, but a distinctive flavor not like strawberry. It was easy.

Gallium Maltolate. I would have never heard of it if it hadn't been for my husband's friend Alex from his deployment years in Afghanistan. Alex was working as a geologist for the US government. My husband was a senior mentor in the AFPAK Hands initiative. In their respective roles, they met through their involvement with Afghani civilians. Over the years, my husband learned that Alex is more than a geologist; he is also a mathematician who founded his own biomedical research company. It was he who told my husband about gallium maltolate's effect on cancer.

After the arrival of the gallium, my husband handed me published papers by the developer of gallium maltolate, a California scientist who knew Alex from their mutual background in minerals and geology. The research and biochemical reasoning for gallium's efficacy against cancer were sound. I started taking it that night. As I waited for my appointments to materialize, I took gallium maltolate daily. Time was critical, and gallium maltolate made sense. Most importantly, I didn't have to sit idly while the insurance companies straightened out our situation.

Chapter III
What Are You, Cancer?

I didn't have many questions for the medical staff at the hospital about my cancer because I knew diddly about cancer. To ask questions intelligently, I have to know something. As soon as I had access to my resources at home, I began to dig into this new subject.

I learned that cancer is not a single disease, it is hundreds of different ones. Even amongst those with the same cancer, the molecular signature[11] for one person's cancer may be different than others. Hence, a treatment plan that helps someone else with adenocarcinoma of lung origin, may not help me.

Cancers vary tremendously, yet they begin when there is a genetic change in the DNA of a cell which produces a mutated cell. What causes this DNA

---

[11] Also called biomarker or molecular marker. It can be used to refine cancer classification and to personalize a patient's therapy. It is typically used to determine how well the body responds to treatment.

mutation? There are many theories. A conservative answer is that it is due to repeated exposure to risk factors which include lifestyle factors, genetics and genetic disorders, exposures to certain viruses or environmental toxins, or high dose radiation and chemotherapy.

Typically, the immune system rids the body of mutated cells because they are diseased. When abnormal cells create mechanisms to survive the immune system, they grow with abandon. Eventually they become a tumor which causes damage to healthy cells. In my case, the cancerous cells which caused the pleural lining of my lung to fill with fluid were destroying one lung and my heart.

My adenocarcinoma started in the glandular epithelial cells which line my lung. These cells produce fluids to keep the lung tissues moist.

No one can say how it started. However, there is a relatively new theory that hypothesizes that a particular type of cell, a cancer stem cell, initiates cancer activity.[12] The origin of the cancer stem cell, of course, is unknown. This cell is thought to be different from other cancer cells in that it has the unique ability to grow quickly, survive, replicate itself and produce other types of cancer cells. Unfortunately, stem cells are resistant to

---

[12] Moselhy. 2015.

chemotherapy and radiation and are considered the cause of tumor recurrence and metastasis.

Some researchers have drawn parallels between cancer stem cell behavior and queen bee behavior[13]. To understand this metaphor, we start by thinking of the cancer stem cell as the queen bee (QB). The QB produces worker bee cancer cells (WB) and drone bee cancer cells (DB). The QB produces many WB and DB cells. WBs & DBs make up the mass of the tumor but they are more fragile than QBs and when exposed to treatment such as radiation or chemotherapy they tend to die.

The QB, however, is difficult to kill.[14] Furthermore, she has the ability to go into a protective slow-cycle state while under stress making it appear as though the cancer has disappeared. Yet later when the QB resumes an active state, the cancer returns. She was fooling everyone. She hadn't gone anywhere and she hadn't died. She was hibernating in plain sight.

The QB produces new QBs and these QBs produce their own populations of WB & DB cells. Either the original or the spawn QBs then migrate to other sites.

---

[13] Tan. 2023.

[14] A cancer stem cell is thought to have the ability to inactivate cytotoxic drugs which makes the stem cell resistant to radiation and chemotherapies.

About one percent of a cancer population is QB cells or stem cells, and 99 percent are WB and DB cells. The QBs are so few, yet so powerful!

When dealing with cancer, various therapies may kill the DBs and the WBs, but not necessarily the QB. This is the incredible foe that we are up against.

Chapter IV
A Cancer Disrupter: Gallium Maltolate

A crucial part of my story and key to my survival is gallium maltolate.

As mentioned earlier, I began taking gallium maltolate the first week after diagnosis. This was the only pro-active thing I could do while all the insurance red-tape was resolved.

Day after day, I awoke to my gallium/water mixture and drank it down. I changed my diet radically to eliminate anything that might interfere with the gallium maltolate. For me this meant no meats, no red nor green vegetables, no coffee, no tomato sauce, no sugar of any form except fruit and occasionally honey, and no alcohol. This left me with fruit, some veggies, rice, noodles, potatoes, eggs, fish, and occasionally chicken. I switched to high alkaline water and tea.

I didn't mind. I wanted to live, even if it meant never eating my favorite foods again.

I started to feel better, but I had no way of knowing whether or not it was working. I had to wait until I had a scan.

About a week after starting gallium maltolate, I had an appointment with my pulmonologist to check on my lung and to determine what we should do about the pleural effusion; primarily whether or not I needed a catheter installed to drain the fluid at regular intervals. I had looked up what this would entail and I was dreading the procedure. Nevertheless, I liked this doctor; he was personable and treated me well. He saw me frequently while I was in the hospital.

At this appointment, he was just as I remembered. He took a bit of time analyzing the x-rays that were taken just prior to the appointment. He listened to my lungs; he looked several times at his computer screen. I sat there, resigned to my fate, and thought about the long day it would be.

Then, he turned to me and said, "I have good news for you and bad news." This did not surprise me. I had heard bad news every day over since this ordeal began.

Then he continued.

"The good news is that the x-ray shows that your lung is almost completely re-inflated and the pleural effusion is nearly resolved."

I was tentatively relieved and asked, "Well then, what is the bad news?"

He looked at me with a sweet smile. "I won't be seeing you anymore."

Yes, I did like him very much, and this bad news made my day!

How was this good news possible? It had to have been the gallium maltolate. I had no other treatment. I resolved then and there to continue with gallium no matter what other treatment was prescribed. Nevertheless, I was still in hot water. For now, I didn't need a tube connected to my lung to get rid of malignant fluid, but I still had the brain lesions to worry about.

Some weeks after this appointment, in September, I went in for my initial Gamma Knife session. The first thing that they did was to take finely-tuned MRI scans to show the neurosurgeon precisely where to aim the gamma knife.

As my neurosurgeon looked over the scans in one room, I waited in the prep room. The anesthesiologist arrived and administered general sedation, which I gratefully accepted. As I slept, the technicians installed a "frame" on my head. They took a large metal cage-like contraption and screwed it into my skull in four places. When it was time for the gamma knife procedure, I would lie down on a test bed, and this cage would be mounted onto a platform on the bed to completely immobilize my head. It was imperative to keep the head still during the procedure.

The drugs wore off and I awoke to the strangest sensation ever. My neck could barely support the weight of the metal cage screwed into my head. I was exploring how this new headpiece felt when the neurosurgeon and two of his techs came into my room with copies of the scans. I was sitting up trying to balance my head while the three of them faced me straight on from the front of the room. The surgeon had a perplexed, suspicious look on his face.

"What happened?" he asked.

"Excuse me?"

"Your brain lesions aren't there. You have a benign growth which should be treated but the malignancies are resolved. What happened?"

I tried to shrug in my normal, *I don't know what you're saying*, type of way but couldn't. Instead I said weakly, "Gallium?"

Either he didn't hear me or he thought I was talking nonsense.

"Now you have to make a decision, do you want to proceed?"

I gave him the most "are you kidding?" look that I could muster although I doubt he could see it. I eagerly replied, "Yes, get rid of it!"

I was still in a fog, but for the first time since my diagnosis, I was happy. Gallium maltolate *was* working.

Gallium maltolate, *why* have you been hiding?

> The oncology world seems largely unaware of gallium maltolate, even though recent papers from multiple research institutions are available. Preclinical research has found gallium maltolate to be effective in animal models of brain cancer,[15] and anecdotal clinical data have shown apparent efficacy for oral gallium maltolate in many advanced cancers (including lymphoma, primary liver cancer, breast cancer, lung cancer, colorectal cancer, bladder cancer, and prostate cancer).[16]

---

[15] Chitambar, 2018.

[16] Bernstein LR, 2013.

Starting in the 1970s, the radioisotope gallium-67 has been used as a diagnostic tool "to locate, stage, and assess the viablity of cancers."[17]

Even though gallium-67 scans have been largely supplanted by newer imaging techniques (such as PET, CT, and MRI), gallium-67 scans are still used for detecting and staging lymphomas, and occasionally other cancers. Also starting in the 1970s, citrated gallium nitrate was investigated as a possible cancer treatment, with some success. During these studies, it was noticed that gallium inhibited the loss of bone mineral from bones, reducing abnormally high calcium levels (hypercalcemia) in cancer patients.[18]

In 1991, a form of gallium called citrated gallium nitrate was approved by the U.S. FDA for the treatment of cancer-related hypercalcemia. The citrated gallium nitrate, though, had to

---

[17] ibid, pp 585-586

[18] Bernstein, 2011.

be administered intravenously (IV), because it was poorly absorbed orally. Unfortunately, IV administration resulted in kidney toxicity when the administration was too rapid. Very slow intravenous infusion was required, usually over at least a five-day period, which made the treatment inconvenient, risky, and expensive.

In response to the need for a safer and more convenient gallium compound, a California scientist, Dr. Lawrence Bernstein, developed a new formulation of gallium, gallium maltolate, that could be safely administered orally and that results in high gallium absorption into the blood. Gallium maltolate is a combination of gallium and maltol, which is a naturally occurring compound found in some plants, including clover, ginseng, licorice, peppers, chicory, and pine. Maltol is also present in many baked foods, as it forms when sugar is heated (it is responsible for the characteristic scent of cotton candy, and gets its name from roasted malt).[19]

---

[19] https://www.gallixa.com/LRB/GaMForCancer.html

Today, gallium maltolate is the preferred form of gallium for therapeutic treatment in clinical studies.

The reason gallium works is conceptually simple. Gallium is a metal[20] that is biochemically similar to the form of iron[21] that is essential for cellular processes in our bodies, such as DNA synthesis and cell division. Healthy cells heavily recycle iron, so they need very little new iron. Cancer cells, however, are greedy consumers of iron. They develop the mechanisms necessary to grab iron faster than normal cells, especially to fuel their rapid reproduction. When gallium is introduced into the bloodstream, it fools the cancer cells into thinking that it is iron. The cancer cells grab the gallium, however, they are unable to use it and become iron-deprived. The cancer cells are no longer able to

---

[20] Atomic number 31, group XIII on the Periodic Table of Elements

[21] ferric ion or Fe^{3+}

synthesize DNA or to divide. This ultimately leads to cell death.

Simple. Easy to administer. Cancer cells seize it with unbridled greed to their own demise.

This was a godsend to me. At the time of this writing, it is still in clinical trials[22] but is available through clinical studies and through a small scattering of integrative oncology practices in the U.S. that offer it as a complementary treatment to cancer, especially brain cancers.

I believe that gallium maltolate was effective for me for two reasons. The first is that I started the gallium maltolate treatment before any conventional treatment. The second is that I adhered to a radical diet. At the time, my instructions were to avoid all reds and greens. That way, I wouldn't be feeding the cancer cells iron. In addition as I mentioned earlier, I eliminated coffee, dairy products, pork, any food that contained processed sugars, and alcohol. It was a difficult diet to follow, but I managed it while I was taking gallium maltolate. I believe all of this worked together.

Gallium maltolate before other treatments plus a restricted diet was the key for me.

---

[22] clinicaltrials.gov

Chapter V

A New Direction

My husband accompanied me to my initial appointment with the oncologist. Our first stop was the billing and insurance office. We were given an overview of the process. It seemed straightforward, but with every paper we signed I began to glimpse the cold business aspect of cancer. It was sobering.

An hour later, we were in the exam room of the oncologist assigned to my case. He was kind and knowledgeable. I had no complaints. He told me that I would receive chemo-therapy infusions after I had finished the Gamma Knife treatment. He repeated what everyone at the hospital had told me. He couldn't fix me.

The silver lining was if they could find a specific genetic mutation, then my care plan would look different and would be less traumatic. But in either case, nothing could be done to get rid of the cancer. At best, they might be able to slow it down. He mentioned palliative care.

I told him about gallium maltolate and gave him a copy of the research. He looked it over and told me that it sounded fine. It would be okay with him if I wanted to take it, especially since I was a terminal patient. It wouldn't interfere with any treatment they would give me. However, as it is not on the FDA list, he couldn't prescribe it and I would have to pay for it out of pocket. I knew this.

I left his office with a vague idea of my treatment, still uncertain about the specifics. I agreed to follow the plan, and while waiting for the results of the genetic test I continued to take gallium maltolate.

―――――

Fast forward several weeks to the day before my third and final Gamma Knife session. The phone rang. It was the oncologist's nurse practitioner.

"I have great news for you!"

"Oh?" I asked.

"Yes, the genetic test results just arrived. You have ALK Positive[23] lung cancer!"

"Oh." I didn't know what this meant. But I was happy she was happy.

―――――――――――――――

[23] Anaplastic lymphoma kinase positive — abbreviated as ALK+

"This is great news. You won't need to have chemo-therapy infusions. All you have to do is take a pill. Just a pill!"

Ah, that is what it meant — just a pill.

Chapter VI

Not Just a Pill

The "pill" that my cheerful nurse practitioner mentioned isn't a simple pill at all. It is a targeted therapy consisting of a family of marvels of innovation, known as *tyrosine kinase inhibitors* (TKIs). These drugs inhibit the action of one or more of 90 tyrosine kinases in the human genome.[24] The theory is that it will block the protein that is causing the uncontrolled growth of the cancerous cells. It will buy me time.

For ALK+ cancer, there are currently five different TKIs available[25]. The goal is to stay on one of the TKIs as long as possible until progression or the side-effects become unbearable. Then, a different TKI is tried.

---

[24] O'Neill

[25] They are in order of generation: crizotinib, alectinib, ceritinib, ensartinib, brigatinib, and lorlatinib

The TKIs are categorized by generation or the order in which they were developed. The later generations have shown a longer progression-free survival rate (PFS). Initially, a patient is typically prescribed an early generation TKI. Eventually when the cancer progresses, the next generation is recommended until there are no more. Lorlatinib, considered to be the most dreaded of the lot, is the newest TKI to date and is currently the last easy FDA-approved therapy for our cancer. After a patient has shown progression on Lorlatinib, the oncologist typically suggests a combination of TKI and chemo infusions or immunotherapy. Some people try to join clinical trials at this point.

My oncology team originally wanted me to start with the first-generation TKI, Crizotinib. My husband and I researched the PFS rate and the most common side-effects. One side-effect which bothered me was that with this drug, I had a 70% chance of severe vision impairment. This was greatly troubling. I didn't want to risk losing my eyesight. My husband and I concluded that this TKI wasn't a good fit for me.[26]

We found a second-generation TKI, Alectinib, that would be a better match. There was still a high probability of severe side-effects, however the PFS rate was higher and it seemed to be a better drug

---

[26] The very low PFS rate was alarming as well.

all-around. My oncology team was receptive to starting me off on Alectinib. It was a go, but I skidded to an early stop due to severe side effects. The full dosage hit me hard. After more research, I found a study in Japan that showed that a half-dosage was equally effective as the full dosage. I made a case for this reduced dosage.

A week after starting Alectinib, I went in for a chest and abdominal scan. The previous scans had been taken in the hospital in late July. I now wanted a baseline scan to document the current state of the cancer.

I wasn't in a hurry to learn the results—who would be? I waited until my next appointment when I learned, incredulously, that all lesions, except the primary one, were no longer visible. Were they gone? Apparently they were! First the brain lesions, now the rest (except the primary). This was clearly a miracle. I thanked God.

I was cautiously relieved. It was not yet Thanksgiving, so I hadn't met my first goal to reach that date. Furthermore, I was struggling with side-effects which left me as exhausted as I had been in early July. I couldn't taste anything and I couldn't tolerate most foods both of which made it a struggle to gain weight[27].

A *h, cancer, you are so cruel! You come and take away all of my fat and tempt me with a lovely figure! But you don't stop. You continue to carve away, leaving me begging for some meat on my bones![28]*

The good news was that I was now free of all lesions except the itsy-bitsy one in my lung, a wee remnant. Yet I was still not out of danger. The Initiator, that horrible Queen Bee stem cell, the One that caused all of the random malignancies to spread and corrupt my innocent body was yet to be extinguished.

I wanted it annihilated.

My oncologist shook his head apologetically. He had nothing to offer that would do that. And, he explained, even if the remnant disappeared, at Stage

---

[27] In the hospital, there was concern that I had developed *cachexia*, which is a wasting syndrome characterized by rapid weight loss that many advanced cancer patients experience. If not dealt with quickly, it may lead to debilitating weakness and the inability to eat, which further compounds the situation. Cancer doesn't just invade a body, it turns the body against itself.

[28] Anonymously me.

IV, I still have cancer cells circulating in my bloodstream which could lodge anywhere in my body at any time. These circulating cancer cells are the reason why I am not and will never be a candidate for surgery as this significantly raises the probability that the cancer cells will land.

In a well-meaning manner, my oncologist's nurse practitioner kept reminding me that although I was still Stage IV, all I have to do is take a pill. And if that stops working, i.e. my cancer starts growing or appears somewhere else, then I take the next pill. The secret is to pray that the cancer does not find a way around the TKI or mutate again, or that the side-effects from the TKI don't become intolerable.

Thanksgiving rolled around and I was still alive. My children plus extras joined us in celebration. Then, I reached Christmas which was incredulous. New Year's Eve was a magical entrance into a new year. My family plus extras gathered together once again and we all celebrated a beautiful evening. Still brain-foggy and struggling with other side-effects, I continued on, month by month until at last, I made it to my first Cancer Anniversary in July 2021! However, by this point I could hardly function at all. The exhaustion was overwhelming.

I went in for a battery of tests, and they found that I had developed severe hemolytic anemia, a rare but known side-effect of Alectinib. The nurse told me to stop the TKI. Then she put me on steroids. A couple of months later, I felt worse than ever. Finally, I stopped taking all drugs to give my body a rest.

That seemed to do it. My energy and my blood levels slowly improved. I started to feel normal.

My original oncologist had by now moved to a new location, and I was assigned to a new one. He and I agreed I would try the next generation TKI, Brigatinib. After two weeks on this, I started to have random episodes of not being able to breath at all — a distinct drowning sensation. I stopped taking it.

This is when the idea to try the third-generation TKI, Lorlatinib, came up. Recent studies[29] had shown that using this TKI as first-line treatment, increases PFS. It crosses the blood/brain barrier and is particularly effective at preventing brain metastasis. Consequently, ALK+ specialists are recommending it strongly, especially for those who have had brain lesions.

Unfortunately, once again the potentially severe side effects were discouraging, chief among them central nervous system (CNS) effects such as change in cognitive function, mood and speech.[30] I had heard many stories about other people's experiences on this drug which further dampened my enthusiasm. Some people developed heart

---

[29] Baba, 2022.

[30] ibid.

problems, other developed severe neuropathy, etc. Further complicating things, I had to be careful taking natural supplements while on Lorlatinib as metabolic consequences were likely.[31]

It was nearly Christmas, the second since my diagnosis. I didn't want to ruin the holidays with a new drug that would put me through the wringer once again. I was feeling a bit normal physically, and I wanted to enjoy this for as long as possible.

I was reluctant to go back on a TKI. However, with each passing day, I risked a resurgence of the cancer. With the support of family and a special group of faithful women, I finally started the TKI and trudged through the first several weeks of side effects. They were mainly cognitive and not pleasant but at least I was neither drowning nor exhausted. It would take over three months to acclimate to it. One can never get used to it entirely. I learned to take it at night, so that the cognitive distortions and disruptions that it causes would mainly affect my dreams. It still impacted my balance, my eyesight,

---

[31] Lorlatinib is primarily metabolized by the enzyme CYP3A in the liver. Therefore one must be careful not to take strong CYP3A inducers or inhibitors. Strong CYP3A inducers such as St. John's Wort, Valerian, and Ginkgo Biloba, may reduce the effectiveness of the drug. On the other hand, natural products including Grapefruit, Ginger, Goldenseal root, Milk Thistle, Kava, Pomegranate juice, Quercetin, Echinacea, and Bergamot are CYP3A inhibitors and may cause a higher concentration of the drug in the bloodstream. Balance must be obtained.

the nerve endings of my fingers and toes, and the foods that I could tolerate.

But as the nurse practitioner told me whenever I saw her, I was very lucky. She was absolutely right. I was lucky and grateful!

Chapter VII
The Face of ALK+

I rack my brain every day, trying to piece together what *caused* this cancer. After searching for answers since my diagnosis, I now realize that modern science simply doesn't know. Many people attempt to dissuade me from pursuing this line of thought because it seems pointless, but I feel that if I can identify what caused this cancer, I have a better chance of figuring out how to turn it off, permanently.

So, I start by asking what does ALK+ look like?

ALK+ is a specific cancer: it is one type of adenocarcinoma NSCLC. It is uncommon and it is one of the many mysteries of the oncology world because no one knows what causes it.

As I have pointed out earlier, I was a very low risk candidate for lung cancer. I've never smoked, and I've lived a healthy lifestyle which included exercise and all the rest that usually comes with this:

a balanced diet full of fruits and vegetables, vitamin supplements, and minimal alcohol consumption. I rarely got sick—never caught the flu nor a cold. My immune system was robust. I had had no exposure to unusual concentrations of toxic substances and there is no history of lung cancer in my family. How did I end up with a Stage IV cancer with no warning?

That is what most ALK+ patients ask.

I found an online organization[32] of patients, researchers, and advocates dedicated to research toward solutions for ALK+. They have an active Facebook group, with over 3500 members worldwide. Through this group, and a couple others, I have gained a wealth of knowledge about ALK+.

For instance, I have learned that my story is very similar for the majority of us. We are in great shape and health. We have never smoked. Over 50% of us are young women (30-50 years old)[33]. We discover we have lung cancer incidentally, and shockingly, 90% of us are initially diagnosed at Stage IV.[34] To be diagnosed with cancer is terrible enough but to be diagnosed with Stage IV is overwhelming. It is

---

[32] alkpositive.org

[33] ibid.

[34] ibid.

frightening news for anyone—especially a young person in great health in the prime of life. It is a death sentence.

One asks, could it have been prevented or caught earlier? No. We have no known method for detecting this cancer unless the tumor is large enough to appear on a routine scan. Living a healthy lifestyle and feeling great is no guarantee that your aren't Stage IV. This is the face of ALK+.

I wanted to clearly see this face, examine its features, and determine where it is most vulnerable. Yet I have no medical or biological training. Trying to understand what ALK+ looks like has been a daunting challenge. I decided to look at it as a *story* featuring ALK+ as the main character:

> Our cancer is the story of a gene called ALK, who won't turn off. ALK makes its first appearance in the embryo in the womb, where much of its job is to provide instructions to form the embryo's central nervous system. ALK's instructions are encoded in receptor tyrosine kinase **proteins.** They help control cell growth, division, death and other processes to develop the central nervous system. The ALK tyrosine kinases chug along merrily doing their job as the embryo grows.

When the systems are ready to go and the embryo is ready to enter the world, ALK essentially turns itself off, for the most part.

The ALK gene from that point doesn't have much to do, or at least we are not sure of what it does. It is a gene without a specifically known purpose. Unfortunately, sometimes a segment of DNA within the ALK gene breaks off. This fragmented segment, all alone and confused suddenly detects another lonely gene, the EML4[35] gene. Recognizing a potential match, they perhaps ask each other, "are we a good fit?" If they answer "yes," then they fuse together and become a new and different gene called EML4-ALK. This new gene is an *oncogene* and has different powers from either ALK or EML4 alone. In the best case scenario, the immune system recognizes the mutated oncogene and destroys it right then and there. However, if it does not, then the *fusion tyrosine kinase proteins are activated and send* signals to cells to grow and divide, but not die. When

---

[35] echinoderm microtube-associated protein-like 4

enough cells have accumulated, they form a tumor.

If the tumor stays localized and is accessible, it can be destroyed by surgical removal or radiation. Once it spreads and metastasizes beyond its point of origin, individual tumors can still be treated by radiation or removal. Generally speaking, however, the cancer cannot be permanently stopped or eradicated. The best that can be done is to try to throttle the action of the fusion tyrosine kinase proteins, thereby cutting off the signaling for uncontrolled growth.

This is what the TKIs do. They rein in the tyrosine kinase proteins by blocking them from sending signals for cell growth. It is a stop-gap measure. It works until our main character, the super oncogene, mutates again and finds another pathway for sending out its signals to grow.

This lung cancer is not your run-of-the-mill life-long smoker's lung cancer. This type of DNA damage is unusual. Of the 85% of lung cancers that are NSCLC, only 4% of those are ALK+. My cancer originated in the glandular cells of my lung which categorizes it as an adenocarcinoma. About 40% of non-small cell lung cancers are adenocarcinoma. So I have the ALK+ mutation of an adenocarcinoma NSCLC type lung cancer. Only about .2 percent (2 out of 1000) lung cancer cases fall into the same category. ALK+ is not something that occurs frequently. There must have been an unusual convergence of factors that brought it about.

What could have caused the breakage of the ALK DNA in the first place? It is not an inherited condition. Is it environmental? Did exposure to radon, freon, asbestos, or lead paint lead to this? Or perhaps chemicals in personal care products such aluminum in deodorants, or dyes and chemicals in shampoos, make-up, lotions, and nail polish are to blame? So much is written about the potential harm of chemicals in plastics and scented candles. What about estrogen? There are studies that have linked estrogen to cancer. Could any of these have been the culprit?

I wonder about things that I might have inhaled such as fiberglass insulation, gasoline fumes, or smoke from wood stoves. Perhaps a bacteria invaded my lung and started the process.

This list of possible causes is so long that it provides little obvious insight. Yet there is a potential common factor. Looking closer at potential causes, I note that they each cause oxidative stress.

> When the body has too many free radicals floating around that have not been neutralized, tissues and cells can be damaged. Oxidative stress has long been implicated in many cancers, especially small-cell lung cancers due to cigarette smoking. However, there is no known connection between oxidative stress (due to environmental factors) and non-small-cell ALK+ cancer. Nevertheless, this line of thought is intriguing.
>
> The two books referenced earlier, emphasized a connection between inflammation and cancer. This correlates to recent studies that also demonstrate "a close interconnection between cancer development and the

clinical, general, and inflammatory status of patients."[36]

Inflammation occurs when proteins called cytokines detect a pathogen (viruses, bacteria, allergens, or other harmful things that enter the body) and call up immune cells to either fight the invaders or heal tissues. Cytokines tell the immune cells where to go and what to do based on type of cytokine. *Anti-inflammatory* cytokines regulate the action of the immune cells preventing inflammation from causing damage.

These cytokines travel either directly into a tissue or via the bloodstream. An abnormally high concentration of cytokines in the blood causes a cytokine storm which may cause excess inflammation and/or autoimmune diseases.

In turn, autoimmune diseases such as Chronic Fatigue Syndrome, lupus, and rheumatic arthritis or viruses such as

---

[36] Mazzella, 2023.

> Epstein-Barr and Herpes Simplex may
> cause *chronic* inflammation.

It is all very complicated with many moving parts and the technical papers are a challenge to read. After connecting some high-level dots, I am reaching the conclusion that the key for my body is maintaining homeostasis. *Balance.* Every part must do its job as it should — neither too aggressively nor too passively — but in perfect balance.

My body is obviously out of whack. Excessive oxidative stress is attacking my cells, trying to throw them off. Meanwhile something somewhere is causing inflammation. The inflammation and the oxidative stress are two actors playing off of one another, gaining strength by doing so, giving cancer free rein.

My immune system is in over-drive in one area when it should be relaxing — but not too much. On the other hand, with respect to the malignant cells it seems to be a bit unresponsive, allowing them to survive. I seek a safe way to give my immune system the tools it needs to ramp up and swiftly pop-off off those mutant cells circulating through my bloodstream, and then quietly go to sleep again, without causing inflammation.

How can my immune system recognize the face of ALK+ to detect and destroy it? No one has an answer. Gallium maltolate may prove to be my most important weapon as amongst its other effects on the body, it also reduces inflammation.

ALK+ LUNG CANCER

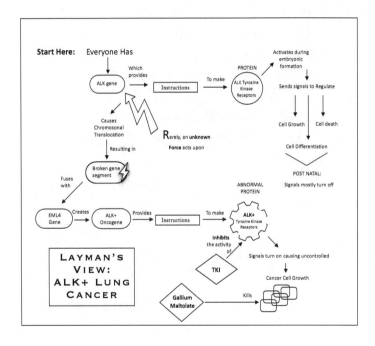

Chapter VIII

All in Good Time

But they that wait upon the LORD shall renew
their strength; they shall mount up with wings
as eagles; they shall run, and not be weary; and
they shall walk, and not faint.

—Isaiah 40:31

So how do we live with terminal cancer? How do we fight the demons of despair that crop up at three in the morning when we can't fall back asleep because of intense foot pain caused by the TKI? How do we convince ourselves to continue to ingest drugs that we know are slowly destroying our organs or our nervous system while we spend our days trying to build up our bodies, pretending that everything is ok? How do we determine if that new pain in our chest is the cancer revitalized or simply a side-effect of the TKI?

By the grace of God, I continue to navigate this landscape, trusting that everything will be okay. That first precarious year was full of jagged rocks and murky skies, but now the cancer is quiet. I won't be lulled into complacency. I continue to try to understand as much as possible about the cancer and search for new ideas, new ways to obliterate it.

I live my life as fully as I can. I am reading three books at a time to work my way through the ridiculous collection that I built up. I am writing, and I am creating art. I am working on my spiritual growth. I constantly add flowers to my gardens. I help with family projects. I visit my adult children.

I can do almost everything I could do pre-cancer, except on the days when I cannot. Those are the days when I realize that my physical body and my cognitive state will forever be affected by both the TKI and the cancer.

Every once in a while, I think back to that hospital stay in the summer of 2020 which heralded tremendous turbulence and uncertainty into my life and the lives of my husband and children.

I think back to my dream of walking the eighty-one miles of the Dales Way in England with my friend, a challenge I was eagerly anticipating. After two years of training, a year of trip planning, and surgeries for new eyesight, I wanted to experience England up close and in focus: her air, her ground, her pathways, her vegetation, her people. I wanted to come home full of vigor and enthusiasm and a new appreciation for our earthly abode.

Yet, if I had gone, I would have not come home alive. I know that now. I had no way of knowing that then.

If the trip hadn't been cancelled by Covid-19, then I would have been somewhere in the remote Yorkshire Dales as my lung collapsed and my heart started to fail. I would have put on a brave face and forced my body to continue on, despite its breakdown. I would have literally walked myself to death in the middle of a foreign land without my family. And what would my friend have done? What does one do when a walking partner suddenly dies in this situation? From the perspective of time, Covid-19 shut down the world and saved my life.

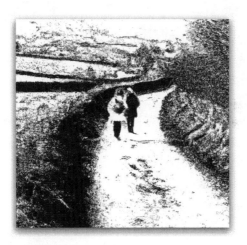

I thought my challenge was to walk the Dales Way. My challenge became cancer.

I n those days Hezekiah was sick and near death. the prophet Isaiah, son of Amoz, went to him and said to him, 'Thus says the Lord: Set your house in order, for you shall die, and not live.'

—2 Kings 20:1

I think back to the emotional impact of that diagnosis which continues to haunt me. What do we do when confronted with a predicament that is so dire that we know that there is not going to be a happy ending? I have always told my children that the test isn't the test, it is your reaction to the test. So my test wasn't the cancer; it was how I reacted to the cancer.

How did I react? Like you might expect. Cancer is such a self-centered disease. It is easy to turn inward to process the gamut of emotions. There's sadness, denial, depression, anger, urgent prayer, rationality, defeat, detachment, hysterical laughter, and tremendous love. The net result was that I turned whole-heartedly to God.

Nevertheless the whole thing was and continues to be emotionally painful not just for me but for my family. My adult children are living their lives. They are each, in their own ways, preparing for the day when I won't be here. They are building close friendship networks and support structures that will take the place of Mom. They pray continuously for my complete recovery. They are protective of me and make decisions with my condition in mind. My husband is an infallible optimist who believes in miracles, thank goodness. He is constantly reaching out to people who might have answers and finding articles about new research and possible cures. His confidence is inspiring.

I have learned to lean heavily on family and friends who keep me from teetering on the tightrope of terminal cancer. They constantly grab hold of me and steady me, urging me forward in the direction I need to go.

This wobbliness, this uncertainty, this heavy reliance on others was hard for me to embrace. Pre-cancer, I faced problems head-on and figured out various solutions: Plans A, B, and C. Post-diagnosis, any plans at all seemed futile.

> *T*hen he turned his face toward the wall and prayed to the Lord, saying 'Remember now, Oh Lord, I pray, how I have walked before You in truth and with a loyal heart, and have done what was good in Your sight.' And Hezekiah wept bitterly.
> —2 Kings 20:2-3

Just as King Hezekiah wept when he learned he was terminal, I too, have shed enough tears to water

Catherine's garden[37]. Like others, I've never relished the idea of being an invalid or of having to be dependent on the health care system. That brief hospital stay in 2020 had a profound impact. For the first time in my life, I was completely vulnerable to the whims of strangers: nurses, doctors, technicians, food deliverers, and most insidiously, the insurance decision-makers. I had to depend on rotating personnel, some of whom I would only see once.

Hooked up to tubes and wires, I couldn't move out of the bed. I couldn't control my food or drink. I had no choice over when medical staff wanted to do something with me. They visited randomly at all hours of the day and night to draw blood or check the tubes or perform some other procedure. There was a camera pointed directly at my bed. I was under constant observation.

I didn't know that I should have packed a bag of necessities. Consequently, I only had my scant summer clothes, my purse, and cell phone, nothing else, not even a phone charger. Until my family could visit, I was completely at the mercy of strangers.

I didn't have Vicks Vapor Rub—the only thing that helped me breathe. I asked a corpsman for some Vicks the first night. He said he would ask about it, but I never saw him again. I asked a nurse.

---

[37] Catherine's future flowers in Heaven will be truly soaked!

She shrugged. I asked another corpsman, this time offering money. He told me he couldn't accept money. No Vicks for me.

When I realized that I didn't have a comb or toothbrush, I asked a nurse for them and offered her money. She came back with a care package that included a toothbrush and paste, but no comb. A day later when she was back on shift, she handed me a black plastic comb that she bought at the exchange. A simple comb—it made me feel human again.

I faced empty hours in the hospital as neither my husband nor my children were allowed to visit but singly for a brief periods of time. Luckily a young intern found a cell phone charger for me. This gave me access to the outside world. I had access to movies and music; I could easily have spent the hours emotionally escaping. But no, I couldn't enjoy any of that. With life so precarious, I couldn't focus on drivel.

It dawned on me that in retrospect, it didn't matter what I ate or drank or how much I exercised throughout my life. I was unable to keep my body healthy. Any pride I had in following a disciplined lifestyle instantly vanished. Despite all my best efforts, I had failed magnificently. I felt as though I had been unceremoniously thrown to the ground to languish: a weak, miserable human being. I failed and I was powerless.

When I returned home, despite its comforts, the words the doctor said to my husband haunted me, "It is very unlikely she'll make it to Thanksgiving."

All of my plans for the future were now moot. The art that I wanted to create, the books I wanted to write were not going to come into being. Those who depended on me would have to find their own ways. My mother, who had early dementia, would never know because it would be too much for her to bear. My family, my friends, would go on to lead their lives as they should. I would barely have enough time to put my things in order so that I wouldn't leave a mess for them to sort through. All of these thoughts were a reprimand to myself for not realizing that I didn't have the time I thought I had. I wasn't afraid of death. I simply wasn't ready to leave my family.

The reprimand wasn't self-pitying; it was humbling. All of it. In this diminished state, I was forced to wrestle one-on-one with humility.

I had to accept the concept: *I, ML, having a name and place in this world, am actually nothing in the overall scheme of things.* Yes, I am a human, with all of the dignity and self-respect that is accorded this station. Yet when it comes down to the essence, I am simply a humble creature with no true power or stature of my own. Anything that I thought I had accomplished wasn't through my own power; it was all a gift. My formerly healthy body, my skills

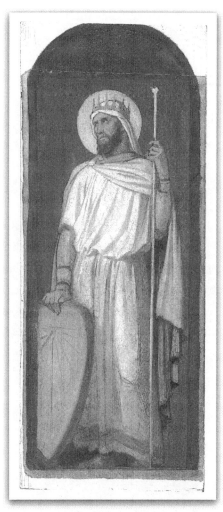

Hezekiah, King of Judah
Hippolyte Flandrin 1856–1863
Oil over pen and brown ink
Metropolitan Museum of Art

in writing or teaching were all a gift. Even my time here on earth was a gift. Somehow, I had failed to comprehend this simple concept at a deep level over the course of my life. Now, facing death, I understood. It isn't about me.

How many times have we been told, *God is in control?* He loves us and wants us to do good things, but He doesn't cede control to us. I have heard this in so many ways and from so many angles throughout my life, and now the clue bird finally landed. God is actually in control. He plopped us, all of us, down onto this earth to accomplish unique missions. He has given each of us something special to do. Often we don't realize this. Onward we struggle, play, and live from one day to the next, hoping that what we are doing is good for us and all, mistakenly thinking that it is up to us to make it happen. Remarkably all along, God is there, trying to remind us that we are in reality here by His grace and we have a reason to be here, apart from our own preconceived, vain-glorious, self-centered feelings that lead us to believe we are here for the good of ourselves.

It became clear that my true test wasn't cancer or how I responded to cancer. My test was a test of my faith. God gave me a prolonged glimpse of the struggle my soul was about to encounter. I could have chosen to be angry with Him or to reject Him when my life was suddenly foreshortened. I chose to try to hear Him, to understand what He wanted from me, with more purpose and clarity than I had ever before attempted.

I thought I had been listening to Him for most of my adult life, but apparently I had not. In those first months after my diagnosis, I was thunderstruck with the realization that I haven't been hearing or perhaps listening to God. If I had, I would have realized long ago that I have never had any power at all here on earth. I was deluding myself my entire life. This was when I began to be lifted up.

*A*nd it happened, before Isaiah had gone out into the middle court, that the word of the Lord came to him, saying, "Return and tell Hezekiah the leader of My people, 'Thus says the Lord, the God of David your father, "I have heard your prayer, I have seen your tears, surely I will heal you. On the third day you shall go up to the house of the Lord. And I will add to your days fifteen years.
— 2 Kings 20:3-5

It has always been God; I was just too arrogant to understand. I had been living a life prioritizing what I thought was important and though I had been seeking God for so long, I never stepped out of my own perspective and shed my biases to recognize Him and His voice.

Being given only three months to live forced me to leave the false security of arrogance. When I did, in a Polaroid flash, the world looked vastly different. The things that I had accumulated, the busy calendars that I had filled, all of my dreams for the future were seen in a new light. I still deeply appreciated the beauty around me, however, I saw everything as fleeting and not strongly attached to me anymore. I felt like a fool for collecting so many projects for the future, and looked upon my possessions as things no longer for my benefit but as a responsibility to leave in good condition for my family.

The people in my life, my family, those who were friends as well as those I knew peripherally assumed a new importance. It became an imperative for me to connect and appreciate a moment with each and every one of them, just for a brief moment if possible, before I died.

It started in the hospital. People streamed in and out of my room, and I wanted to know who they were. They were happy to stop for a moment and tell me little snippets of their stories. There were so many fascinating ones! I heard about a romantic Covid-19 marriage between two residents straight out of medical school in one of the rooms of the campus buildings. They couldn't invite guests, but their parents managed to be present. I learned about a young woman's family who had a flower farm that supplied most of the flowers in Southern California. One young corpsman wanted to buy some land in the South and build his own house. He had no idea how to start the process of looking for land. We talked about online resources such as Zillow, and how to research land possibilities.

One of my nurses, in her mid-forties, had had cancer when she was in her twenties. She reminisced that even though the chemo was terrible, and it was the worst six-months of her life, the hardest part was when she lost all of her hair. Standing by my bed, she laughed and shook her head of gorgeous blond hair. It had all come back, and she was even able to have children.

Another active-duty nurse, who had school-age children, was about to undergo medical tests which she dreaded. If they turned out positive, she would be discharged from the Navy. If that happened, she didn't know how she would manage.

One nurse, who came in late one night told me her story. She and her husband settled in the U.S. when they were young adults. They had good jobs and their children were thriving. They had found happiness here. I was glad to hear her tell me this. Then she explained that although she is content, she had not been spared her share of pain. This is when she spoke to me about a terrible tragedy her family endured almost exactly a year before.

As she told her story, I was surprised that she could remain radiant and serene while recounting harrowing details.

When I asked how this is so, she explained that her peace draws from her unwavering trust in God. She told me to trust God; He would heal me.

She asked if I wanted her to pray over me. I nodded. Without hesitation, she enveloped me in strong arms. Her hands against my back were incredibly warm. This warmth lingered.

Before the nurse left, she mentioned 2nd Kings in the Bible. She couldn't remember the exact passage or the details off-hand, but she told me that it had to do with one of the Kings and healing. Without knowing a thing about 2nd Kings, I asked her if it concerned Hezekiah.[38] To my astonishment, she said it did. She told me she'd find it for me.

Many hours later at the end of her shift, she slipped into my room and without saying a word, handed me a scrap of paper. On it was written 2 Kings 20. It was as though she handed me a golden key.

The personnel continued to flit in and out of my room, and some I would only see one time in my life, but they were willing to take a moment to share a part of themselves with me. Their stories touched my heart and gave me strength.

---

[38] Why did Hezekiah pop into my mind? I hadn't read the Book of Kings. I do, however, have a great-great-great-great-great grandfather from Sudbury, Massachusetts named Hezekiah Walker. Throughout my life, I have been intrigued by his name.

As soon as family and friends found out about my situation, a rush of prayers flowed from my phone. I have tried to find the words that describe the feeling that surrounded me once the prayers began, but I haven't yet. I simply knew it would all work out in the end. Even if I died before Christmas, it would still be fine.

Through the procedures and tests, I learned to slip into an alternative state of mind which enabled me to pray to Our Lady continuously and offer up my pain for the souls in purgatory. I couldn't think clearly enough to make my petitions more specific, but I hoped at least one soul benefited.

I left the hospital a greatly bruised and chastised human being. I had never felt so low in my life.

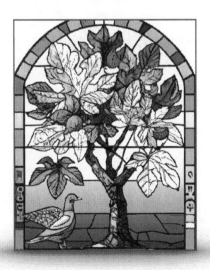

T hen Isaiah said, 'Take a lump of figs," So
  they took and laid it on the boil, and he
recovered.

—2 Kings 20:7

I returned home to a lush garden where the fig
trees were laden with fruit. I love figs and have been
known to eat gobs of them in one sitting. Yet now I
couldn't taste them and the sight of them did not fill
me with joy. They were just there. I had no appetite
for figs or anything else.

The people in my life, however, wouldn't let me
languish. They appeared with food including such
favorites as home-made quiches, grilled chicken,
shepherd's pie, chicken pot pie, breads, and French
fries. At first I wanted to say "No thank you—I can
take care of things myself." Then I realized I
couldn't. I humbly accepted all that was offered.
That was very hard. I was in a new place as I
gratefully accepted these gifts.

There were so many flowers! One arrangement,
a cheerful potted mums, had a place of prominence
on our family room coffee table. After its bloom, I
planted it in the front garden. Today it flowers
abundantly in the early autumn reminding me of
my friend and of all of the prayers that she and her
family have prayed for me.

One brother, Rob, learned that I could tolerate cashew nuts, an important source of nutrients. I have yet to run out of cashews, unsalted.

And then there was Chuck, who out of the blue banded together with his fiancé (now wife), and daughter to cook dinners for us for an entire year. This grill-master knew my diet was ridiculous, yet night after night he created delicious meals that I could eat. How does one thank such generosity?

The flowers, the gifts, and the food were all love letters. They were prayers in tangible form that filled me with hope, popping up here and there, always unexpectedly and yet when I most needed them, especially in that first year and a half during which I was navigating medications, scans and debilitating side-effects. I only had a few good hours per day and I was existing in a perpetual state of fog. I didn't trust that things would ever get better but was grateful to still be alive and that the cancer was quiet.

When I switched medications to the targeted therapy, Lorlatinib, whose long list of side-effects was daunting, something in me rebelled. I didn't want to take this. My bible study group, The Holy Mamas, heard my tale of woe. They insisted I take the medication.[39] I continued to express concern. As a surprise, they organized a "Twelve Days of

---

[39] Many of them are nurses!

Christmas Recovery Rally" to cheer me on and bolster my spirits.

Inspired by the carol, *The Twelve Days of Christmas*, the rally started on Christmas Day and continued throughout Twelvetide. Each day, one of the Holy Mamas, sometimes with their families, appeared at my door with a gift, a message and prayer.

This was the first time I experienced a group of people praying for my well-being as the Holy Mamas did that season. Surely their prayers and actions helped flip a switch. I took the new pill and pushed through the side-effects. Before long, my body became acclimated. I could think and see again and all was well. It was evident after about a month that I would be able to tolerate it which meant that the cancer would continue to be throttled, and I had more time. This was the gift these women gave to me.

All of these experiences and all of the people who have prayed for me have taught me the power of prayer. Sometimes we ask God for help for ourselves, sometimes for others. Sometimes we just want to say, *thank you*. No matter the reason, it is an expression of our faith in Him. The results are often astonishing.

I now have a deep desire to know God. I want to talk to Him and hear His voice through prayer.[40] I am learning to look for this connection in the quiet of my mind, in the depth of my heart. And intriguingly, I believe His voice is music.

> *A*sk, and it shall be given you; seek, and ye shall find; knock, and it shall be opened unto you.
>
> Matthew 7:7

When I can't hear Him, it is probably because I have driven myself into a fog, obstructing my vision.[41] Yes, He is there; he is perpetually there. My hope is that I will always continue to strive to hear His answers and to trust that He has placed them within my reach. I must keep asking and seeking. I must keep remembering: He wants to help us, and He gives us everything we need to succeed.

And I must remember, *it isn't about me.*

This is how I live with terminal cancer.

---

[40] My favorite discussion on prayer, is *Time for God* by Jacques Philippe.

[41] Why do I need vision to hear God? I don't know, but the two seem intertwined.

*T*he spirit of humility is sweeter than
honey, and those who nourish
themselves with this honey produce
sweet fruit.

— St. Anthony of Padua

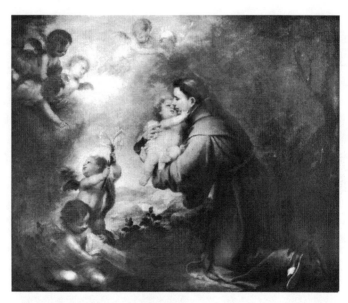

Saint Anthony of Padua with the Christ Child by Murillo, ca. 1670-1680. Location
unknown. Destroyed or disappeared in Berlin in May 1945, in the Friedrichshain
flak tower fire.

Chapter IX
Serendipity & Miracles

A *nd Hezekiah said to Isaiah, 'What is the sign that the Lord shall heal me and that I shall go up to the house of the Lord on the third day?'*

—2 Kings 20:8

I was strolling through a consignment shop awhile ago when I heard two women conversing loudly about a clock that one of them was holding.

One said, "But what would you do with it?

The other replied, "The same as any other clock!"

"But you can't read it. Everything's backwards. Time doesn't go backwards."

"I don't care! I'm buying it." The second lady said.

I thought this was the funniest exchange. It reminded me of an incident long ago when I was a young girl. I was in the kitchen chatting with my mother. One of us must have asked what the time was. We glanced simultaneously at the old General Electric kitchen clock above the door to the dining room. The moment we looked at the clock, the second hand inexplicably moved counterclockwise for about a minute. Just as suddenly as it went backwards, it resumed its clockwise movement. My mother and I stared at it, perplexed, before bursting into nervous laughter. Not knowing anything about how electricity works, we concluded that the current must have somehow reversed. That was all. My father, a physicist, came in to see what the commotion was about. When we told him what had happened and our theory as to why, he rolled his eyes and chimed in with great authority that it was the house ghost.

It was a moment of merriment in our family.

Since my Stage IV diagnosis, I spend much time reflecting on the links between my past and the present. I consider incidents throughout my life that lead to where I am today. I try to understand what the patterns mean in the overall scheme of things, and where they in turn will lead. A clock from my childhood that once misbehaved by turning counterclockwise for a minute…the backward clock forever running counterclockwise...the slip of paper handed to me upon which was written 2 Kings 20, the story of a king who witnessed time going backwards. Why?

These three stories have a common element: time reversal. However, my two fleeting stories were just that—*fleeting*. Whereas Hezekiah's story remains relevant today. For three years, I have mulled over it.

King Hezekiah, a righteous man, grew gravely ill. God healed him and gave him an additional fifteen years of life. However, Hezekiah wanted a sign from God confirming this good news.

*T*hen Isaiah said, This is the sign to you from the Lord that the Lord will do the thing which He has spoken: shall the shadow go forward ten degrees or go backward ten degrees?

— 2 Kings 20:9-10

Isaiah gave King Hezekiah a choice. Did he want time to *proceed* or *recede*?

*A*nd Hezekiah answered, "it is an easy thing for the shadow to go down ten degrees; no, but let the shadow go backward ten degrees."

Hezekiah knew that it was normal for time to move forward; he wanted to see it move backwards.

> *S*o Isaiah the prophet cried out to the Lord and He brought the shadow ten degrees backward, by which it had gone down on the sundial of Ahaz.[42]
>
> —2 Kings 20:11

Isaiah asked God to grant Hezekiah this miracle and God responded. The shadow went backwards ten degrees. What could this possibly have looked like for Isaiah and Hezekiah?

I couldn't find a definitive explanation for how time-keeping was accomplished in those ancient days. Experts don't agree on the actual mechanism or design of the sundial referenced in the Bible.

Upon careful examination of the description amongst different translations of the Bible, I noticed that variations of the wording of the passage provide clues. In the King James Version, the word "degrees" is used as units of time. In other translations, "steps" is used. With respect to time moving forward, "go down" or "decline" is typically found. With respect to describing backward time movement, we find the verb phrases "turn backward," "go backward," and "retreat."

---

[42] Ahaz was the father of Hezekiah. The sundial of Ahaz is presumably a sundial that had been constructed during the time of Ahaz.

The miracle itself is written as "He brought the shadow on the stairway back ten steps by which it had gone down on the *stairway* of Ahaz," "made the shadow retreat the ten steps it had descended on the *staircase to the terrace* of Ahaz," and "He brought the shadow ten degrees backward, by which it had gone down on the *sundial* of Ahaz." Finally, the structure used for tracking time is described variously as a shadow on a "*stairway of Ahaz*," "*staircase to the terrace of Ahaz*," the "*dial of Ahaz*," and the "*sundial of Ahaz*."

We know that Ahaz is the father of Hezekiah. By reference, we can conclude that this time-keeping mechanism was built by Ahaz before Hezekiah ascended to the throne. Considering these words and their variants, a picture does emerge.

We can infer that the sundial was imposing because the miracle created a spectacle. A small sundial couldn't have that effect. It had to have been visible to many people including Hezekiah on his deathbed. A pillar which cast a shadow on a set of steps in the middle of the courtyard would have been seen by many. If those steps became longer nearer the bottom, then the lengthening shadows that cast upon them would effectively measure each hour. Conceivably, each step could mark about a degree of sun position.

If the shadow on the steps went up the stairs, instead of down, then observers could conclude the sun unnaturally reversed its movement or time went backward. How was it possible that the shadow moved backward? Various critical thinkers through the years have postulated that it was a clever illusion caused by unusual cloud movement, an abnormal refraction of the sun's rays, an eclipse, or an earthquake. The Church Fathers and other scholars have concluded that the effect was local and not celestial. However science isn't settled on the matter.[43]

Time moving backwards in any age is an intriguing concept. It captures our imaginations and is brought to life in many creative forms.[44] For King Hezekiah and those around him, it was an unambiguous and powerful manifestation of God's glory and presence in their lives. When people near and far heard of the miracle, they flocked to Hezekiah. The same instinct propels people today to travel great lengths to visit sites where miracles occur such as the shrines of Our Lady of Walsingham, Our Lady of Lourdes, and Apparition Hill at Medjugorje.

---

[43] Biblio-archeologists are exploring the possibility that this event was celestial and felt around the world. Using evidence in pottery shards dating to the time of Hezekiah which suggest that the earth's geo-magnetic field spiked suddenly "followed by an immediate and dramatic field-weakening…The current research suggests that Hezekiah's spike *was* worldwide." https://armstronginstitute.org/306-geomagnetism-hezekiahs-seals-and-the-sun-turned-back

[44] "Hello Sweetie!" Carved in rock: *Riversong's timeless greeting to Dr. Who*

Yet there is another wrinkle in Hezekiah's story. If one continues reading Isaiah's words beyond the time reversal miracle, one may begin to question Hezekiah's true test. Was his illness a test of faith? Or was his true test his reaction to the miracle granted to him? How did he react when God reversed time for him?

> *A*t that time Merodachbaladan, the son of Baladan, king of Babylon, sent letters and a present to Hezekiah: for he had heard that he had been sick, and was recovered.
>
> And Hezekiah was pleased with them, and showed them the house of his treasures, the silver, and the gold, the spices and the precious ointment, and all of his armour, and all that was found in his treasures: there was nothing in his house, nor in all his dominion, that Hezekiah did not show them.
>
> —Isaiah 39:1-2

After the miracle, Hezekiah joyfully received visitors including envoys from far-off Babylon who expressed great interest in the King's wealth. From the accounts, Hezekiah generously showed all of his possessions to the strangers.

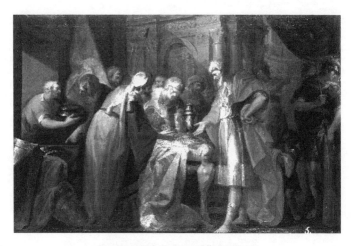

King Hezekiah Showing Off His Wealth
Vicente López Portaña 1789, oil
Museo de Bellas Artes de Valencia (wikicommons)

*T*hen Isaiah the prophet went to King Hezekiah, and said to him, "What did these men say, and from where did they come to you?" So Hezekiah said, "They came to me from a far country, from Babylon."

And he said, "What have they seen in your house?" So Hezekiah answered, "They have seen all that is in my house: there is nothing among my treasures that I have not shown them."

—Isaiah 39:3-4

From these lines, we can imagine that after the sun miracle, Hezekiah was exuberant. And in the delirium of his joy, he lost perspective and became proud. This arrogance led him to imprudently show off his possessions.

I can relate to this temptation. I survived past the death time frame estimated by my doctor, and afterwards my first and then second anniversary of diagnosis. I have begun to feel like myself again which makes me gloriously happy. If I had a singing voice that wasn't embarrassing, I would sing from the rooftops. But luckily, the people who surround me, the interactions with my ALK+ group, and the constant physical reminders that the TKI is a double-edged sword keep me grounded in humility. I try mightily to remember every day that *but for the grace of God…*

Isaiah tried to warn Hezekiah, but evidently he didn't hear.

> *T*hen Isaiah said to Hezekiah, "Hear the word of the Lord of Hosts:'Behold, the days are coming when all that is in your house, and what your fathers have accumulated until this day, shall be carried to Babylon, nothing shall be left,' says the Lord. 'And they shall take away some of your sons who will descend from you, whom you will beget: and they shall be eunuchs in the palace of the king of Babylon,'"
>
> —Isaiah 39:5

Hezekiah won the battle, but due to his pride lost his kingdom.

> *So Hezekiah said to Isaiah, "The word of the Lord which you have spoken is good!" For he said, "At least there will be peace and truth in my day."*
>
> —Isaiah 39:6

Yet, he was relieved that he would continue to reign over Judah in peace until he died and was reportedly unconcerned about the fate of his descendants. How can this be right? Who in good faith lives in serenity while knowingly cursing their descendants?

I come full circle to connect the dots. I consider what has captured my attention: Hezekiah's sun miracle when time apparently reverses (a miracle that continues to draw attention thousands of years later); an old electric kitchen clock with a second hand that turns counterclockwise for one minute and never again; and a backward clock that materializes randomly, just out of reach.

Serendipity or coincidence? How does God reach us humans, especially when we are struggling or enmeshed in fog? Hezekiah knew his answer came directly from God. He had a prophet who was well-connected. We, however, in our current age, don't have that luxury and if we did, would probably not trust the messenger.

I believe that these three incidents are pieces in the puzzle of my life that help me begin to see a bigger picture. After everything that I have been through since July 2020, patterns show me that God's hand has been manifest in all that has happened. In all of the little serendipitous details I have experienced, in people he has put in my path, and in words that I have heard that pierce my heart, He is telling me that He is indeed here. Like Peter walking on the stormy waters, I must reach out to Him.

I have learned that we are called to be humble. I am able to love more deeply than I thought possible. This is what we are capable of and what we should strive for. Ideally, we understand this before something catastrophic happens, before we are *forever Stage IV*. We learn to live our lives loving God and one another, not just once a week but throughout all of our days. We learn that we have been placed in this world to do God's will, to follow our unique mission using the gifts He has given us. We trust that He will guide us if we reach out to Him.

I live with a ticking time bomb in my lung and bits of it circulating through my bloodstream. I don't know when or if it will go off again. It doesn't matter. I shall live my life while striving to do what I believe I am supposed to do. Being diagnosed with Stage IV cancer was a supreme test of my faith; living with Stage IV cancer is now an opportunity to deepen and share my faith while still on Earth. I have the same mission to complete as before but now with a clearer understanding and realization that God has been by my side my entire life. I wish I had known earlier that I have always had what I needed for this mission, but it's never too late. I can move forward with strength and courage.

By the grace of God, I have yet a field of boulders to scamper over before He calls me home. This I shall do joyfully while keeping my eyes on Heaven.

No more clouds. I can see clearly for the first time in my life.

—⁂—

S eek ye first the kingdom of God, and his
righteousness; and all these things shall
be added unto you.

—Matthew 6:33

Acknowledgements

Thank you, dear readers, for this time together.

Bill, husband-extraordinaire, you have showered me with love from the moment we met; I wouldn't want to be here without you. Thank you for being you and for your eclectic and colorful set of friends!

Heartfelt thanks to my daughter Anneliese, chief editor and cover designer, for encouraging me and constantly sending good thoughts my way.

Grateful thanks to my son Nathan, a man of action and compassion, who boldly saved my life and continues to be an inspiration to me.

To my daughter Genevieve, who always pops in with surprises, I thank her for her strength, generosity, and loving heart.

I thank my resilient brother, Joseph, cancer survivor, for his kindness and for keeping me on my toes with witty repartee.

To my mother, TVH, a tribute to her sparkle.

I thank my bother and sister-in-law, Rob and Ellen, for their uplifting support and endless supply of cashews, unsalted.

Much gratitude to Dr. Larry Bernstein, developer of gallium maltolate; Dr. Bo Zhao, my oncologist; Dr. Javier Amadeo, my neurosurgeon; Dr. Charles R. Kersh, my radiation oncologist; Dr. Michael Hamilton, my eye surgeon, Dr. Dari Lane, my PCP; NP-C Miriam New, and all of the medical staff for giving me and others the opportunity to live meaningful lives despite cancer. Thank you for the additional time.

Thank you to the many people who kept me going that first year especially: Georgetta and Jill Deal, Al and Michele Pendleton, Chuck and Alexa McLean, Alex and Natasha Chaihorsky, Gwen and Jim Sturdy, St. Bede Holy Mamas Heather Clemens, Elizabeth Berquist (and family), Becky Carvajal, Kathy Gillespie (and family), Liz Hansen, Catherine White, and Jennifer Gillette.

For those who have been placed in my path, who help complete the puzzle, even though I may not have mentioned you by name, you are in my heart and I thank you!

Ad Majorem Dei Gloriam

Glossary of Acronyms

- ALK+ : Anaplastic Lymphoma Kinase positive
- CFS : Chronic Fatigue Syndrome
- CNS : Central nervous system
- CT scan : computed tomography
- EKG : electro-cardiogram
- EML4 : echinoderm microtube-associated protein-like 4
- FDA : Federal Drug Administration
- DB : drone bee
- ICU : Intensive Care Unit
- NSCLC : Non-small cell lung cancer.
- MRI : magnetic resonance imaging
- PET scan : positron emission tomography
- PFS : progression-free survival
- QB : queen bee
- TKI: tyrosine kinase inhibitor
- WB : worker bee

References

Baba, Keisuke, and Yasushi Goto. "Lorlatinib as a treatment for ALK-positive lung cancer." *Future Oncology* (London, England) vol. 18,24 (2022): 2745-2766. doi:10.2217/fon-2022-0184

Bernstein LR. "Gallium, therapeutic effects," in *Encyclopedia of Metalloproteins*, Kretsinger RH, Uversky VN, and Permyakov EA, eds., 2013, pp. 823-835, Springer, New York; https://www.gallixa.com/LRB/GaMForCancer.html

Bernstein, LR, van der Hoeven JJ, Boer RO. "Hepatocellular Carcinoma Detection by Gallium Scan and Subsequent Treatment by Gallium Maltolate: Rationale and Case Study." *Anticancer Agents Med Chem*. Vol. 11, no. 6, pp 585-90, 2011, doi: 10.2174/187152011796011046. PMID: 21554205.

Bernstein, LR. "Mechanisms of therapeutic activity for gallium." *Pharmacol Rev*. Vol 50, no. 4, pp 665-82, 1998, PMID: 9860806.

Chitambar CR, Al-Gizawiy MM, Alhajala HS, Pechman KR, Wereley JP, Wujek R, Clark PA, Kuo JS, Antholine WE, Schmainda KM. "Gallium maltolate disrupts tumor iron metabolism and retards the growth of glioblastoma by inhibiting mitochondrial function and ribonucleotide reductase." *Molecular Cancer Therapeutics*, 2018, DOI: 10.1158/1535-7163.MCT-17-1009

Mazzella, Antonio, Elena Maiolino, Patrick Maisonneuve, Mauro Loi, and Marco Alifano. "Systemic Inflammation and Lung Cancer: Is It a Real Paradigm? Prognostic Value of Inflammatory Indexes in Patients with Resected Non-Small-Cell Lung Cancer" *Cancers* 15, no. 6, 2023, p. 1854, https://doi.org/10.3390/cancers15061854

McLelland, Jane. *How to Starve Cancer ... without Starving Yourself: One Woman's Extraordinary True Story of Survival, Courage and a Discovery That Could Transform Millions of Lives.* Agenor Publishing, 2018.

Moselhy, Jim et al. "Natural Products That Target Cancer Stem Cells." *Anticancer research* vol. 35,11, 2015, pp. 5773-88.

Philippe, Jacques. *Time for God.* Scepter Publishers, Inc. 1992.

Seyfried, T.N., MD. "Cancer as a Metabolic Disease" *Nutrition Metabolism* (London) 2010; 7:7.

Stegall, Jonathan, MD. *Cancer Secrets: An Integrative Oncologist Reveals How You Can Defeat Cancer Using the Best of Modern Medicine and Alternative Therapies.* Published by the author, 2020.

Tan, Swee, MD. *Gillieo McIndoe Research Institute,* Wellington, New Zealand gmri.org.nz, accessed April 2023.

Further Reading

Bosch-Barrera, Joaquim et al. "Response of brain
metastasis from lung cancer patients to an oral
nutraceutical product containing silibinin."
Oncotarget vol. 7,22 (2016): 32006-14. doi:10.18632/
oncotarget.7900

Elisia, Ingrid, and Gerald Krystal. "The Pros and Cons of
Low Carbohydrate and Ketogenic Diets in the
Prevention and Treatment of Cancer." *Frontiers in
nutrition* vol. 8 634845. 25 Feb. 2021, doi:10.3389/
fnut.2021.634845

Haider, Mohamed et al. "The Potential Role of Sildenafil
in Cancer Management through EPR
Augmentation." *Journal of personalized medicine* vol.
11,6 585. 21 Jun. 2021, doi:10.3390/jpm11060585

Hanahan, Douglas, and Robert A Weinberg. "Hallmarks
of cancer: the next generation." *Cell* vol. 144,5
(2011): 646-74. doi:10.1016/j.cell.2011.02.013

Haskins, Christopher et al. "Low Carbohydrate Diets in
Cancer Therapeutics: Current Evidence." *Frontiers
in nutrition* vol. 8 662952. 25 Nov. 2021, doi:10.3389/
fnut.2021.662952

Hocking, Ashleigh et al. "The Safety and Exploration of the Pharmacokinetics of Intrapleural Liposomal Curcumin." *International journal of nanomedicine* vol. 15 943-952. 11 Feb. 2020, doi:10.2147/IJN.S237536

Keats, Theodore et al. "The Rationale for Repurposing Sildenafil for Lung Cancer Treatment." *Anti-cancer agents in medicinal chemistry* vol. 18,3 (2018): 367-374. doi:10.2174/1871520617666171103100959

Raclariu-Manolică, Ancuţa Cristina et al. "Authentication of milk thistle commercial products using UHPLC-QTOF-ESI + MS metabolomics and DNA metabarcoding." *BMC complementary medicine and therapies* vol. 23,1 257. 21 Jul. 2023, doi:10.1186/s12906-023-04091-9

Sudhesh Dev, Sareshma et al. "Receptor Tyrosine Kinases and Their Signaling Pathways as Therapeutic Targets of Curcumin in Cancer." *Frontiers in pharmacology* vol. 12 772510. 15 Nov. 2021, doi:10.3389/fphar.2021.772510

Talib, Wamidh H et al. "Melatonin in Cancer Treatment: Current Knowledge and Future Opportunities." *Molecules* (Basel, Switzerland) vol. 26,9 2506. 25 Apr. 2021, doi:10.3390/molecules26092506

Tang, Wenfang et al. "TNM stages inversely correlate with the age at diagnosis in ALK-positive lung cancer." *Translational lung cancer research* vol. 8,2 (2019): 144-154. doi:10.21037/tlcr.2019.03.07

I *see clearly with the interior eye,*
That the sweet God loves with a pure love
the creature that He has created, and has
a hatred for nothing but sin, which is more
opposed to Him than can be thought or
imagined.

— St. Catherine of Genoa

About the Author

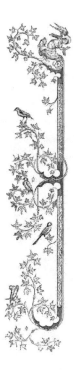

Millie Lintell was diagnosed with Stage IV lung cancer in the middle of the Covid-19 pandemic. Her case was dire and doctors had little hope that she would survive. Before packing it in and saying good-bye, she turned to the excellent people all around her and asked for help. An outpouring of support, love, prayers, and God's grace have given her what she needed to get over this boulder. This little book is her account of her journey.

Made in the USA
Columbia, SC
03 November 2023